Table of Contents

Lymphedema is swelling in various areas of your body that happens when something affects your lymphatic system. Your lymphatic system collects excess fluid, proteins and toxins from your cells and tissues and returns them to your bloodstream.

When your lymphatic system doesn't work well, your body accumulates fluid and may begin to swell. The swelling typically affects your arms and legs, but it can affect other areas of your body, too. Lymphedema also increases your risk of developing an infection where you have the condition.

This can happen after certain surgeries or because you have certain medical conditions or genetic conditions. You may develop lymphedema spontaneously, meaning it happens for no known reason.

Lymphedema symptoms may be mild, causing minor swelling and discomfort. Sometimes, however, lymphedema may cause significant swelling that can be painful and cause skin issues such as infections and wounds. Healthcare providers can't cure lymphedema, but they do have treatments to reduce lymphedema swelling and discomfort. There are also many things you can do to limit the impact lymphedema may have on your quality of life.

BREAKFAST

1. Breakfast Burrito

Prep Time: 20 Minutes

Cook Time: 35 Minutes

Servings: 8

Ingredients

- Sara's Herb Cream Cheese
- Sara's Roasted Plum Tomatoes
- Sara's Salad Greens Mixture
- Sara's Scrambled Eggs
- 4 twelve-inch spinach tortillas
- Extra-virgin olive oil
- 8 ounces smoked salmon
- 8 tablespoons alfalfa sprouts
- 1 small bunch basil, minced, for garnish
- 4 scallions, white part only, julienned, for garnish
- 1/2 small red onion, thinly sliced, for garnish

Instructions

1. Prepare the herb cream cheese, roasted plum tomatoes, and salad-greens mixture. Prepare the scrambled eggs, and keep them warm.

2. Heat a grill pan over medium-high heat on the stove. Using a pastry brush, brush tortillas with olive oil. Grill each tortilla lightly on one side for no longer than 1 minute (the tortillas should be soft and easy to roll). Transfer tortillas, grilled side down, to work surface.

3. Divide herb cream cheese among the tortillas, spreading evenly and leaving a 1-inch border.

4. Divide the smoked salmon, scrambled eggs, and salad-green mixture evenly among tortillas. Top with alfalfa sprouts.

5. Fold in opposite sides of one tortilla, and roll it up; repeat with remaining tortillas. Slice each burrito in half diagonally, transfer to a platter, and garnish with roasted plum tomatoes, basil, scallions, and red onion.

Prep Time: 15 Minutes

Cook Time: 15 Minutes

Servings: 4

Ingredients

- 1 pint strawberries, rinsed, hulled, and thinly sliced
- 1 to 2 tablespoons dark-brown sugar, firmly packed
- 1 3/4 cups milk
- 1/4 teaspoon salt
- 2 cups quick-cooking oats
- 1 tablespoon sour cream

Instructions

1. In a small bowl, toss 1 pint strawberries, rinsed, hulled, and thinly sliced, with 1 to 2 tablespoons firmly packed dark-brown sugar. Let sit at least 5 minutes to bring out the juices.
2. In a medium saucepan over medium heat, warm 1 3/4 cups water, 1 3/4 cups milk, and 1/4 teaspoon salt.

Stir in 2 cups quick-cooking oats; cook, stirring occasionally, until thick and creamy, 5 to 6 minutes.

3. Ladle oatmeal into bowls. Top each serving with 1 tablespoon sour cream and some of the strawberries; sprinkle with brown sugar.

Prep Time: 15 Minutes

Cook Time: 15 Minutes

Servings: 4

Ingredients

- 2 medium red potatoes, scrubbed and cut into 1-inch pieces
- 3 tablespoons canola oil
- 1/2 teaspoon ground cumin
- 1 jalapeno, seeded and finely diced
- 3 scallions, cut into 1/4-inch slices (reserve 1 for garnish)
- 8 ounces cherry tomatoes, halved
- 1 can (15 ounces) black beans, drained and rinsed
- 2 teaspoons nutritional yeast seasoning
- 1 package (8 ounces) plain, pasteurized organic tempeh, crumbled
- 1 medium avocado, coarsely chopped
- Coarse salt and freshly ground black pepper

Instructions

1. Bring potatoes to a boil in a pot of salted water. Cook until knife-tender, about 6 minutes. Drain and set aside.

2. Heat 2 tablespoons oil in a large saucepan over medium-high heat. Add cumin and cook until fragrant, about 30 seconds. Add potatoes and cook, stirring occasionally, until golden, 5 to 7 minutes. Transfer to a bowl; set aside.

3. Heat remaining oil over medium heat. Cook jalapeno, scallions, tomatoes, beans, yeast, and tempeh, stirring, until tomatoes begin to break down, 5 to 7 minutes. Add potatoes and cook until heatedthrough. Remove pan from heat and gently stir in avocado. Season with salt and pepper. Garnish with reserved scallion.

Prep Time: 30 Minutes

Cook Time: 45 Minutes

Servings: 6

Ingredients

- Coarse salt and freshly ground pepper
- 3/4 pound celery root, peeled and cut into 1/2-inch pieces (2 cups)
- 3/4 pound Yukon Gold potatoes, peeled and cut into 1/2-inch pieces (2 cups)
- 3/4 pound sweet potatoes, peeled and cut into 1/2-inch pieces (2 cups)
- 1/4 cup extra-virgin olive oil, divided
- 1 onion, diced
- 2 small firm, sweet apples, peeled and cut into 1/2-inch pieces (2 1/2 cups)
- 1/4 cup roughly chopped fresh sage leaves

Instructions

1. Bring a medium pot of water to a boil, and generously season with salt. Add celery root, and simmer 3 minutes. Add potatoes and sweet potatoes, and simmer vegetables 2 minutes more. Drain well, and spread vegetables on a rimmed baking sheet. Let cool 15 minutes.

2. Heat 2 tablespoons oil in a large (preferably cast-iron) skillet over medium-high heat, and cook onions until translucent and just beginning to color, about 2 minutes. Add remaining 2 tablespoons oil, the apples, and vegetables; season with salt and pepper. Stir to combine, then press into a single layer using a spatula. Cook, undisturbed, 2 minutes. Stir, and repeat process until vegetables are very tender and beginning to caramelize, 8 to 10 minutes more. Remove from heat. Stir in sage, and season with salt and pepper.

Prep Time: 30 Minutes

Cook Time: 45 Minutes

Servings: 6

Ingredients

- 1 cup homemade applesauce
- 1/4 cup raw honey, or pure maple syrup
- 2 large eggs, room temperature
- 2 Tbsps unrefined coconut oil, melted
- 1/2 cup natural peanut butter, or almond butter
- 1 tsp vanilla extract
- 1/2 cup oat flour (blended/ground oats)
- 1 tsp baking soda
- 1/2 tsp baking powder
- 1 tsp ground cinnamon
- 1/4 tsp ground cloves
- 1/4 tsp nutmeg
- tiny pinch of sea salt
- 1/4 cup chopped pecans
- 1/4 cup golden raisins, or dried cranberries

Instructions

1. Preheat your oven to 350 degrees f. Lightly spray two 12-mini muffin molds with nonstick spray.
2. In a medium bowl, stir together the applesauce, honey, eggs, coconut oil, peanut butter and vanilla.
3. In a separate bowl, whisk your oat flour, baking powder, baking soda, cinnamon, cloves, nutmeg, and sea salt.
4. Add this mixture to the bowl with the wet ingredients and whisk just until combined.
5. Do not overmix.
6. Stir in your pecans and raisins.
7. Spoon this batter into the prepared muffin cups filling each 3/4 to the top.
8. Bake for 15-18 minutes, or until the tops are golden brown and a toothpick inserted into the center comes out clean.
9. Remove from the oven and let them cool completely on the wire rack.

Prep Time: 10 Minutes

Cook Time: 35 Minutes

Servings: 4

Ingredients

- 2 medium russet potatoes, scrubbed
- 2 Tbsps avocado oil, or olive oil
- 4 slices nitrate-free bacon
- 4 large eggs
- 1/3 cup shredded cheddar cheese
- 2 Tbsps sliced chives
- sea salt and fresh ground black pepper, to taste

Instructions

1. Arrange your oven rack so that it's right in the center of the oven, then preheat your oven to 400 degrees f.
2. After thoroughly washing; pierce those potatoes with a fork a few times, then rub or brush with oil and rub it all over.
3. Place the potatoes directly onto the center oven rack.

4. Bake for 30-40 minutes or just until potatoes are tender when pierced with a knife.

5. Remove from the oven and allow them to cool a bit.

6. Once ready to handle, slice each potato in half lengthwise and scoop out the flesh as shown. Reserve flesh for another use.

7. Place your potato boats into a baking dish and season them with sea salt and pepper.

8. Add one slice of bacon, shredded cheese, and gently crack an egg into each one as shown.

9. Return your potatoes to the hot oven and bake for about 15 minutes, or just until egg whites just set and yolks are still runny.

10. Garnish with fresh chopped chives and ground black pepper and enjoy!

Prep Time: 10 Minutes

Cook Time: 35 Minutes

Servings: 4

Ingredients

- 4 (16-ounce) mason jars
- 2 large bananas, cut on half then sliced lengthways
- 1 cup fresh berries
- 1 cup plain or vanilla Greek yogurt
- 1 cup granola
- 4 scoops homemade berry sorbet
- 2 Tbsps melted dark chocolate

For the Berry Sorbet:

- 2 1/2 cups frozen mixed berries
- 2 tsp lemon juice, freshly squeezed
- 2 Tbsps raw honey
- 2-3 Tbsp warm water, only as needed

Instructions

1. To make your berry sorbet: Place all the sorbet ingredients in a high speed blender or food processor. Process until smooth and creamy, stopping to scrape the sides a few times.
2. Transfer the sorbet mixture to a freezer-safe container, cover and freeze for at least 2 hours before serving.
3. To assemble the banana split jars: Place half of the banana slices into each mason jar nicely as shown.
4. Divide the yogurt and granola equally among the bowls, then top with s scoop of sorbet and fresh berries as shown.
5. Drizzle melted chocolate and serve immediately.

Prep Time: 10 Minutes

Cook Time: 35 Minutes

Servings: 4

Ingredients

- 2 medium-large avocados
- 4 small eggs
- Topping ideas:
- feta cheese, crumbled
- bell pepper, diced
- nitrate-free bacon, chopped
- organic corn chopped from the cob
- green onions, sliced
- pitted olives, sliced
- sea salt, to taste
- fresh ground black pepper, to taste

Instructions

1. Preheat your oven to 400 degrees f.

2. Cut each avocado in half and carefully remove the pits.

3. Then, using an ice cream scoop or spoon, take some of the flesh out to create a bigger space for your egg and toppings (chop the avocado and use as topping too, or mash with lime to eat on the side).

4. Gently crack an egg into each avocado cup.

5. Sprinkle with your favorite toppings, then transfer the avocado halves to a baking sheet.

6. Season with sea salt and fresh ground black pepper to taste.

7. Bake in your preheated oven for 12-15 minutes, or until the eggs are cooked to your liking.

Prep Time: 10 Minutes

Cook Time: 35 Minutes

Servings: 4

Ingredients

- 4 large eggs
- 1 tsp apple cider vinegar
- 1 large ripe avocado
- juice of half a lemon
- 2 cups cooked quinoa
- 1.5 cups cherry or grape tomatoes, halved
- 1/3 cup crumbled cheese of choice, such as parmesan, cotija, or feta
- 4 thin slices of nitrate free bacon, cooked and crumbled
- 1 jalapeño, thinly sliced
- 1/2 tsp chili flakes
- sea salt and fresh ground black pepper

Instructions

1. Fill a pan with about 2 inches deep with water and bring it to a steady gentle simmer.
2. Add in the vinegar and once simmering use a wooden spoon to make a twirl into the water.
3. Gently tip the egg into the water. Simmer for about 3-5 minutes, or until done to your liking.
4. Lift the egg out with a slotted spoon and drain it on a paper towel.
5. Meanwhile, mash the avocado with a fork and squeeze fresh lemon juice over to keep it green and fresh. Season with a pinch of sea salt and pepper.
6. Divide the quinoa among 4 meal prep containers, then top each bowl with equal amounts of: cherry tomatoes, mashed avocado, poached egg, crumbled cheese and crispy crumbled bacon.
7. Garnish with jalapeño slices, fresh ground black pepper and chili flakes, then sprinkle with sea salt to taste.
8. Enjoy immediately, OR; seal and refrigerate for up to 3 days for food prep.

Prep Time: 10 Minutes

Cook Time: 35 Minutes

Servings: 4

Ingredients

- 12 large eggs
- 12 thin slices nitrate free bacon
- sea salt and fresh ground black pepper, to taste

Instructions

1. Preheat your oven to 400 degrees f.
2. Arrange one slice of bacon into each slot of a 12 count muffin pan, wrapping it around to line the sides as shown.
3. Gently crack an egg into each as shown.
4. Repeat with remaining bacon and eggs.
5. Sprinkle with sea salt and fresh ground black pepper.
6. Bake for about 12-15 minutes or until bacon is crisp and eggs are cooked to your liking.

7. if you like your yolks runny, then place your bacon arrangement alone in your preheated oven for 8-9 minutes first, then remove from oven, gently crack eggs into each, then return to the oven for 4-6 minutes until yolks are to your liking.

8. Serve immediately, OR place into meal prep containers and refrigerate for up to 3-4 days.

11. Happy Rainbowls

Prep Time: 30 Minutes

Cook Time: 45 Minutes

Servings: 4

Ingredients

- 1/2 cup dry quinoa, rinsed well
- 1 cup stock or broth
- 1 red bell pepper, sliced
- 1 large carrot, peeled and sliced
- 1 summer squash, chopped
- 1 cup broccoli florets
- 1 cup shredded purple cabbage
- 1 cup chicken or turkey leftover, chopped or shredded
- 2 green onions, thinly sliced

To Serve:

- toasted sesame oil, coconut aminos

Instructions

1. Rinse quinoa using a fine mesh strainer, then drain it completely.
2. Place your rinsed quinoa in a small/medium pot with broth. Bring to a boil, then reduce the heat to low.
3. Top the pot with a strainer and arrange your bell pepper, carrot, summer squash, broccoli, and cabbage on top as shown in the video.
4. Cover the pot and simmer where the broth is just bubbling for about 15 minutes until the liquid has been completely absorbed. Check by pulling back the quinoa with a fork to see if any liquid remains.
5. Turn off the heat and let sit with the lid on to steam for 5 minutes, then fluff the quinoa with a fork. Add sea salt and pepper to taste.
6. Remove your pot from the heat and allow everything to cool until ready to handle.
7. Divide your quinoa equally between 2 serving bowls.
8. Arrange your steamed veggies and cooked leftover chicken on top of the quinoa.
9. Garnish with chopped green onions.
10. Serve with a drizzle of sesame oil and coconut aminos if desired.
11. Enjoy!

Prep Time: 30 Minutes

Cook Time: 45 Minutes

Servings: 4

Ingredients

- 2 Tbsps avocado oil or olive oil
- 1 medium onion, diced
- 4 ribs celery, diced
- 3 medium carrots, peeled and diced
- 3 fresh garlic cloves, minced
- 15oz jar of diced tomatoes with juices
- 15oz can white beans, drained and rinsed well
- 1 cup uncooked barley
- 4 cups water, vegetable broth, or bone broth
- 2 bay leaves
- sea salt and pepper, to taste

Instructions

1- Set a large heavy-bottomed stock pot over medium-high heat. Once hot, add in your oil, diced onion, celery, and carrots. Saute for 3-5 minutes until the veggies are tender.

2- Give the barley a quick rinse under the water using a fine mesh sieve before cooking, to wash away any dust.

3- Add in your rinsed barley, tomatoes with their juices, beans, water or broth, and bay leaves. Bring to a boil, and then reduce the heat and cover. Simmer for at least 20 minutes.

4- Add in the garlic, and season to your taste with sea salt and pepper. Simmer for another 5-10 minutes.

5- Carefully remove bay leaves before eating.(You may opt to leave the bay leaf in as a garnish for presentation. Just remember it should be removed before consuming.)

6- Enjoy your stew while hot.

7- Leftovers store well in the fridge for up to 5 days.

Prep Time: 30 Minutes

Cook Time: 45 Minutes

Servings: 6

Ingredients

- 1 Tbsp avocado oil or olive oil
- 1 large onion, diced
- 1 zucchini, cut in half lengthwise and sliced
- 1 summer squash, cut in half lengthwise and sliced
- 2 bell peppers, seeded and diced
- 2 Tbsps homemade taco seasoning, divided
- 1-1/2 lbs lean ground beef
- 1 x 15oz can black beans, drained rinsed
- 1 x 8 oz jar green or red salsa
- 1 clove of fresh garlic, minced
- 3 green onions, sliced
- a handful of fresh parsley or cilantro, chopped
- corn chips if desired

Instructions

1. Heat the oil in a large skillet over medium-high heat.

2. Sauté the onion, zucchini, squash, and peppers for about 4 minutes. Stir in half of the taco seasoning and continue to cook for 1 minute longer. Set veggies aside on a plate.

3. Add your ground beef into the skillet and cook while breaking it up with a wooden spoon until no longer pink. Drain any excess grease. Sprinkle cooked beef with remaining taco seasoning, then stir to incorporate.

4. Stir in the beans, salsa, and minced garlic, then continue to cook for 3 minutes.

5. Return the veggies back into the skillet, stir to heat, then garnish with green onions, freshly chopped herbs, and chips as desired.

6. Enjoy!

Prep Time: 15 Minutes

Cook Time: 45 Minutes

Servings: 4

Ingredients

- 2 1/2 teaspoons dried tarragon
- 2 teaspoons grated lemon zest
- 1 1/4 teaspoons coarse salt
- 1/4 teaspoon ground pepper
- 4 bone-in chicken breast halves
- 1/3 cup low-fat plain yogurt
- 2 teaspoons plus 1 tablespoon olive oil
- 3 teaspoons fresh lemon juice
- 3 plum tomatoes, coarsely chopped
- 4 scallions, thinly sliced
- 6 ounces mesclun (about 6 cups)

Instructions

1. Preheat oven to 425 degrees. Rub tarragon, 1 teaspoon lemon zest, 3/4 teaspoon salt, and 1/4 teaspoon

pepper under chicken skin. Place on a rimmed baking sheet; roast until cooked through, about 30 minutes.

2. In a large bowl, whisk together yogurt, 2 teaspoons olive oil, remaining 1 teaspoon lemon zest, 1 teaspoon fresh lemon juice, and remaining 1/2 teaspoon salt.

3. Remove and discard skin and bones from chicken; thinly slice meat lengthwise. Add to bowl along with tomatoes and scallions; toss to combine.

4. In a separate bowl, whisk together remaining 2 teaspoons lemon juice and 1 tablespoon olive oil. Add mesclun; toss to coat. Divide among plates; spoon chicken mixture on top.

Prep Time: 30 Minutes

Cook Time: 45 Minutes

Servings: 4

Ingredients

- 2 skinless salmon fillets (about 8 ounces each)
- coarse salt and ground pepper
- 2 heads Boston lettuce
- Steamed Green Beans
- Rosemary Potatoes
- 4 plum tomatoes
- 3 Hard-Cooked Eggs for Salmon Nicoise Salad
- 1 medium red onion
- 1 jar or tin (2.8 ounces) anchovy fillets, drained (optional)
- 1/4 cup Kalamata (or black) olives
- Dijon Vinaigrette
- Lemon-Herb Bread

Instructions

1. In a 5-quart pot, bring 1/2 inch water to a boil; add salt and twelve ounces (four to five) new potatoes. Cover; cook, turning occasionally, until tender, 14 to 16 minutes.

2. With a slotted spoon, transfer potatoes to a bowl. Set aside to cool. Add eight ounces green beans to the pot of boiling water. Cover; cook, stirring occasionally, until tender, 4 to 6 minutes. Remove with a slotted spoon. Rinse under cool water, and set aside.

3. Fill a deep skillet with 1/4 inch water. Season salmon on both sides with salt and pepper; place in skillet. Bring water to a gentle simmer; cover, and cook until salmon is opaque throughout, 10 to 12 minutes. Transfer to a plate; flake with a fork, and let cool.

4. While salmon is cooking, tear lettuce into pieces, quarter potatoes and tomatoes, peel and quarter eggs, and thinly slice onion.

5. On a large platter (or four serving plates), arrange lettuce, salmon, green beans, potatoes, eggs, tomatoes, onion, anchovies (if using), and olives. Serve with Dijon Vinaigrette on the side.

Prep Time: 15 Minutes

Cook Time: 30 Minutes

Servings: 4

Ingredients

- One 10-ounce loaf ciabatta, halved horizontally and soft interior removed
- 1/3 cup Pesto for Prosciutto Panini
- Extra-virgin olive oil
- 1/3 pound Prosciutto de Parma, thinly sliced
- Tapenade for Prosciutto and Pesto Panini, optional
- 1/4 pound fontina cheese, thinly sliced
- 1/2 cup baby arugula or basil, optional
- Coarse salt and freshly ground pepper

Instructions

1. Preheat a grill pan over medium-high heat or a panini press.
2. Spread one cut side of ciabatta with the pesto and the other with olive oil. Layer one side of ciabatta with

prosciutto, tapenade, if desired, red pepper, and arugula or basil, if desired; top with cheese. Drizzle with olive oil and season with salt and pepper. Top with remaining bread.

3. Brush top and bottom of the sandwich with olive oil. Place on grill pan and weight top of sandwich with a heavy skillet or a foil-wrapped brick. If using a panini press, grill according to manufacturer's instructions. Grill 3 to 4 minutes on first side, turn, weight down, and continue cooking until sandwich is golden and cheese is melted, 3 to 4 minutes.

4. Cut sandwich into quarters. Serve immediately.

Prep Time: 10 Minutes

Cook Time: 20 Minutes

Servings: 6

Ingredients

- 1 tablespoon oil
- 1 cup onion, diced
- 1 cup carrot, diced
- 1 cup celery, diced
- 1 tablespoon garlic, minced/grated
- 1 tablespoon ginger, minced/grated
- 1 teaspoon cumin
- 1 teaspoon coriander
- 1/2 teaspoon turmeric
- 1/4 teaspoon cayenne (optional)
- 3 cups vegetable broth (or chicken broth)
- 1 (14 ounce) can coconut milk
- 2 pounds zucchini, diced
- 1 tablespoon fish sauce
- 1 tablespoon lemon juice
- salt and pepper to taste

- 2 tablespoons cilantro, chopped

Instructions

1. Heat the oil in a large sauce over medium-high heat, add the onion, carrot and celery and cook until tender, about 10 minutes.
2. Add the garlic, ginger, cumin, coriander, turmeric, and cayenne and cook, mixing, until fragrant, about a minute.
3. Add the broth, coconut milk and zucchini, bring to a boil, reduce the heat and simmer until the zucchini is tender, about 10 minutes.
4. Optionally puree some or all of the soup with a stick blender, in a food processor or a blender and return to the pan.
5. Add the fish sauce and lemon juice before seasoning with salt and pepper to taste.
6. Mix in the cilantro and enjoy!

Prep Time: 15 Minutes

Cook Time: 2hrs 20 Minutes

Servings: 4

Ingredients

- 1 tablespoon oil
- 1 pound beef, cut into bite sized pieces
- 1 onion, diced
- 2 cloves garlic, chopped
- 4 cups beef broth
- 1 can Irish stout (or 2 cups beef broth)
- 1 teaspoon rosemary, chopped
- 1 teaspoon thyme, chopped
- 2 bay leaves
- 2 medium white potatoes, cut into bite sized pieces
- 3 carrots, cut into bite sized pieces
- 1 tablespoon Worcestershire sauce
- 1 tablespoon fish sauce (optiaonal)
- salt and pepper to taste

Instructions

1. Cook the beef in the oil in a large sauce pan over medium-high heat until browned on all sides before setting aside and draining off all but 1 tablespoon of the grease.

2. Add the onion and cook until tender, about 5 minutes.

3. Add the garlic and cook unitl fragrant, about a mintute.

4. Add 1/2 cup of the broth and deglaze the pan by scraping any brown bits up from the bottom of the pan as the broth sizzles before adding the remaining broth, stout, rosemary, thyme and bay leaves.

5. Bring to a boil, reduce the heat and simmer, covered, until the beef is almost falling apart tender, about 2-3 hour, OR transfer to a preheated 350F/180C oven and roast, covered, until the beef is tender, about 2-3 hours, OR transfer to a slow cooker and cook on low for 6-10 hours or on high for 3-5 hours.

6. Add the potatoes and carrots and cook until tender, about 15 minuites.

7. Add the Worcestershire sauce and fish sauce before seasoning with salt and pepepr to taste.

Prep Time: 15 Minutes

Cook Time: 30 Minutes

Servings: 4

Ingredients

- 1-1/2 lbs boneless skinless chicken, chopped into bite sized pieces
- 2 Tbsps fajita or taco seasoning
- 1 Tbsp avocado oil, or olive oil
- 3 large bell peppers, chopped
- 1 large onion, chopped
- 1/2 cup chicken bone broth
- 2 oz organic cream cheese or full fat Greek yogurt
- 1/4 cup freshly shredded cheddar
- 2 jalapeños, seeded and diced
- 2 green onions, sliced

Instructions

1. Place the chicken in a bowl together with the seasonings and oil. Toss thoroughly to combine, then allow it to marinate for 15 minutes or so.
2. Preheat a large skillet over medium high heat.
3. Cook the chicken in batches, about 8 minutes per batch, or until cooked through and golden brown.
4. Set your cooked chicken aside on a plate.
5. In the same skillet add your bell peppers and onion, and stir fry for 2-3 minutes. Remove from skillet and det aside.
6. Add the broth into the skillet and stir through the bottom to deglaze. Add in the cream cheese and cheddar, and continuously stir or whisk to create a smooth sauce.
7. Return your cooked chicken and veggies to the skillet and into the sauce and allow it to cook for a minute longer, just to heat everything up.
8. Top with jalapeño, green onions, and an extra sprinkle of grated cheese if desired.
9. Enjoy!

Prep Time: 15 Minutes

Cook Time: 30 Minutes

Servings: 4

Ingredients

- 1 large head of broccoli, cut into bite-sized florets
- 16 oz nitrate-free sausage, sliced
- 2 Tbsps avocado oil
- 1 Tbsp Italian seasoning (or any of your favorite seasoning blends)
- 1 tsp red pepper flakes, or to taste
- sea salt and freshly ground pepper, to taste
- 1/2 cup cheddar cheese, shredded

Instructions

1. Preheat your oven to 400 degrees f. and line a large sheet pan with parchment paper.
2. Add the broccoli florets and sausage to your prepared pan.

3. Drizzle with avocado oil spray and sprinkle with all of the seasonings.

4. Use your clean hands to combine everything really well.

5. Roast for 15-18 minutes, or until the broccoli is tender-crisp to your liking.

6. Sprinkle with shredded cheese then roast for 2 additional minutes, or until the cheese is melted.

7. Enjoy!

21. N Santa Fe Inspired Sweet Potatoes

Prep Time: 15 Minutes

Cook Time: 30 Minutes

Servings: 4

Ingredients

- 4 medium sweet potatoes, scrubbed and pat dry
- 2 Tbsps avocado oil or olive oil, divided
- 1 large onion, diced
- 4 fresh garlic cloves, pressed
- 1 lb ground turkey or chicken
- 1 x 8oz jar salsa

Optional topping ideas:

- plain Greek yogurt
- cherry tomatoes, chopped
- avocado, diced
- green onions, sliced
- sliced fresh jalapeno
- freshly grated Colby Jack cheese

Instructions

1. Preheat your oven to 400 degrees f. and line a medium sheet pan with parchment paper for easy cleanup.
2. Place your sweet potatoes on the prepared sheet pan, lightly rub each of them using 1 Tablespoon oil total, then poke them a few times with a fork.
3. Roast for 35-45 minutes, or until fork-tender. Carefully remove from the oven and allow them to cool just until safe to handle.
4. Meanwhile, preheat the remaining 1 Tablespoon of oil in a large skillet over medium heat. Saute the onion for 3 minutes, then add in the garlic and saute for another minute or so.
5. Add in the ground meat and cook, mincing the meat with your spatula as it browns. Once the meat is brown and cooked through, stir in the salsa and remove from heat.
6. Slice each sweet potato in half lengthwise to create a pocket. Season the inside flesh with sea salt and pepper then gently fluff with a fork, while still keeping the roasted skin intact.

7. Spoon in the meat mixture as desired, then top with a dollop of yogurt, cherry tomatoes, avocado, jalapeno, and green onions.

8. If desired sprinkle the top with a bit of freshly grated cheese then place your stuffed potatoes back into the oven just until nice and melty.

9. Enjoy!

Prep Time: 20 Minutes

Cook Time: 40 Minutes

Servings: 6

Ingredients

- 1 pork tenderloin, about 1–1/2 pounds, cut into big pieces
- 1 large yellow or white onion, diced
- 4 cloves of fresh garlic, pressed
- 4 poblano peppers, seeded and diced
- 1 x 16 oz jar of salsa verde (I like the "Siete" brand)
- 1 x 4 oz jar of mild diced green chilis
- 1 x 13.5 oz can of full-fat unsweetened coconut milk
- zest of 2 fresh limes
- 4 limes, juiced
- 2 tsps ground cumin
- sea salt and ground black pepper, to taste
- 2 x 15-ounce cans of cannellini beans, drained and rinsed

Topping ideas:

- green onions, sliced
- fresh cilantro, to serve
- chopped avocado
- jalapeno, sliced
- lime wedges
- cooked brown rice, to serve

Instructions

1. Place all of the pork ingredients except for the beans in your crockpot.
2. Cook on HIGH for 3-4 hours or on LOW for 7-8 hours. I prefer cooking on the low setting if you have time to produce more tender pork.
3. Once the time is up, remove the pork and shred using 2 forks. Return the
4. meat to the crockpot and stir in the beans.
5. Cook on HIGH for 20 minutes more just to heat through.
6. Serve your pork chili Verde with toppings of choice.
7. Enjoy!

Prep Time: 20 Minutes

Cook Time: 40 Minutes

Servings: 4

Ingredients

- 1-1/2 lbs boneless, skinless chicken thighs
- 4 sweet peppers, sliced
- 4 vine tomatoes, chopped into large bite-sized pieces
- 4 medium garden cucumbers or 1 English cucumber, coarsely chopped
- 1 small red onion, sliced
- 1/2 cup crumbled feta cheese
- 1 cup pitted kalamata olives

Greek marinade:

- 1/3 cup extra-virgin olive oil
- 1/4 cup red wine vinegar
- 2 Tbsps pure maple syrup or raw honey
- 1 Tbsp dried oregano
- 1 tsp garlic powder
- 1 tsp sea salt

- 1/2 tsp freshly ground pepper

Instructions

1. Chop your chicken into small bite-sized pieces and place it in a shallow dish.
2. In a small jar add all the marinade ingredients and shake vigorously to combine. Or simply whisk your marinade together really well until emulsified.
3. Pour half of your marinade over the chicken and toss to coat. Allow chicken to marinate for at least 10-20 minutes on the counter, OR overnight in the refrigerator.
4. Reserve the remaining half of the marinade, (untouched by raw chicken) to drizzle over your meal prep bowls just before serving.
5. Heat a large skillet over medium-high heat.
6. Add in your marinated chicken and cook until golden brown and cooked through around 10 minutes.
7. Meanwhile, chop your veggies as desired for your bowls.
8. Once the chicken is done, allow it to cool then divide it equally into your meal prep bowls.

9. Next add the peppers, tomatoes, cucumbers, feta cheese, and olives to your bowls.

10. Drizzle with the remaining (untouched) marinade as desired.

11. Keep refrigerated for up to 3 days.

12. Enjoy!

Prep Time: 25 Minutes

Cook Time: 55 Minutes

Servings: 6

Ingredients

- 2 Tbsps olive oil or avocado oil
- 5 fresh garlic cloves, peeled and thinly sliced
- 2 x 15 oz cannellini beans, drained and rinsed if using canned
- sea salt and ground pepper, to taste
- 1 x 16 oz jar artichoke hearts, drained and chopped
- 6 cups roughly chopped fresh spinach
- 1 Tbsp freshly squeezed lemon juice
- 1/2 cup grated parmesan or pecorino romano

Optional:

- crushed red pepper flakes, to taste

Instructions

1. Heat your oil in a large skillet over medium-high heat.

2. Add in the garlic and saute for 30 seconds, stirring continuously.

3. Stir in your cannellini beans, season lightly with sea salt and pepper then cook for 4-6 minutes.

4. Next, add in the artichoke hearts, spinach, and fresh lemon juice, then cook for 2-3 minutes, or until the spinach is wilted.

5. Sprinkle everything with parmesan cheese and enjoy immediately while hot.

Prep Time: 25 Minutes

Cook Time: 55 Minutes

Servings: 6

Ingredients

- 2 Tbsps olive oil or avocado oil, divided
- 1-1/2 lbs boneless skinless chicken breast, cut into small thin strips
- 16 oz mini carrots or baby carrots, quartered lengthwise
- Sesame sauce:
- 1/3 cup coconut aminos, tamari, Braggs liquid aminos, or low sodium soy sauce
- 3 Tbsps raw honey
- 2 Tbsps apple cider vinegar
- 3 tsp toasted sesame oil
- 2 fresh garlic cloves, minced
- 1.5" knob fresh ginger, minced
- 1 Tbsp cornstarch or Arrowroot powder
- 2 tsps toasted sesame seeds, or to taste

To serve:

- 3 cups cooked brown rice, quinoa, or cauliflower rice

Instructions

1. Heat 1 Tablespoon of oil in a large skillet over medium heat. Add the chicken in a few separate smaller batches and cook until golden-brown and cooked through. Cooking in smaller batches helps to get your chicken to that nice golden brown.
2. Remove cooked chicken from the pan and set it aside.
3. In the same skillet, add the remaining 1 Tablespoon of oil and sauté carrots until tender-crisp, stirring constantly. About 4 minutes.
4. In a small bowl, whisk all the sesame sauce ingredients together really well.
5. While your skillet is still on the heat with the carrots, add in all the cooked chicken and pour in your sesame sauce.
6. Simmer everything over medium-low heat for 2-3 minutes, stirring frequently. Once your sauce has thickened a bit and carrots are tender, then it's ready!

7. Divide your chicken & carrots equally and serve each portion over 1/2 cup of cooked brown rice, quinoa, or cauliflower rice.

8. Enjoy while hot!

Prep Time: 25 Minutes

Cook Time: 55 Minutes

Servings: 4

Ingredients

Pineapple Salsa:

- 2 cups fresh pineapple, diced small
- 3 fresh green onions, finely sliced
- 1 red chili pepper, seeded and chopped
- juice of 1 fresh lime

Chicken:

- 1-1/2 lbs boneless skinless chicken breasts or thighs, cut into bite-size pieces
- sea salt and ground black pepper, to taste
- 2 Tbsps avocado oil or olive oil, divided to cook the chicken in batches

Serving:

- 2 cups cooked brown rice, quinoa, or cauliflower rice
- large bunch of fresh cilantro, chopped

- a handful of unsweetened dried coconut flakes
- fresh lime wedges

Pineapple sauce:

- 1/3 cup coconut aminos, Braggs liquid aminos, low sodium soy sauce, or tamari
- 1/3 cup fresh pineapple juice
- 1 Tbsp raw honey or pure maple syrup
- 1/3 cup tomato puree
- 1 Tbsp Arrowroot powder, or cornstarch
- 2 fresh garlic cloves, pressed
- 1 Tbsp grated fresh ginger
- 1 tsp toasted sesame seeds

Instructions

1. Prepare your pineapple salsa ingredients then combine everything in a glass bowl and set aside in the fridge.
2. Chop the chicken, pat dry with a paper towel, and season lightly with sea salt and pepper.
3. Preheat your oil in a large skillet over medium heat. Add in the chicken and cook in several batches to

avoid overcrowding the pan. This helps to get those nice crisp edges and tender insides.

4. Saute until nicely golden brown and cooked through.

5. In a large bowl, whisk all of your pineapple sauce ingredients together really well.

6. Once the chicken is finished cooking place it all back into the hot skillet over medium heat then drizzle in your pineapple sauce. Stir frequently with a wooden spoon and allow the sauce to thicken a bit and to completely coat the chicken.

7. Serve your chicken with sauce over cooked brown rice, quinoa, or cauliflower rice, then top with a big spoonful of your fresh pineapple salsa, fresh cilantro, limes wedges, and shredded coconut.

8. Enjoy!

Prep Time: 25 Minutes

Cook Time: 55 Minutes

Servings: 4

Ingredients

- 1-1/2 lbs boneless skinless chicken breasts or thighs, cut into bite-sized pieces
- sea salt and ground black pepper, to taste
- 2 Tbsps GF flour, Arrowroot powder, or cornstarch
- 3 Tbsps clarified butter or ghee, divided
- 1 cup chicken bone broth
- 4 cloves fresh garlic, pressed
- a handful of fresh parsley, minced
- a handful of fresh oregano, minced

Instructions

1. Chop your chicken and place it into a bowl. Sprinkle with sea salt, pepper to taste, and then sprinkle with the flour or cornstarch and stir to coat well.

2. Preheat a large skillet over medium heat. Add 1 tablespoon of ghee/butter and 1/3 of the chicken with some space in between the pieces. Cook the chicken until golden brown and cooked through, then set aside. Repeat with the remaining ghee/butter and chicken. We want to do this step in small batches so the chicken can crisp up and get nicely golden.

3. Once all the chicken bites are done, place them all together into the skillet.

4. Stir in the broth, garlic, and fresh herbs. Continue to cook over medium heat, for 2 minutes, or until hot and the garlic releases its flavor.

5. Serve chicken immediately over rice or quinoa.

6. Leftovers will keep 4 days in the refrigerator or up to 1 month in the freezer.

7. Enjoy!

Prep Time: 25 Minutes

Cook Time: 1hrs 15 Minutes

Servings: 4

Ingredients

- 1 Tbsp avocado oil or olive oil
- 1 Tbsp clarified butter or ghee
- 4 boneless skinless chicken breasts
- sea salt and freshly ground black pepper to taste
- 4 Tbsps GF flour or Arrowroot powder
- 4 slices nitrate-free bacon, chopped
- 2 shallots, small diced
- 3 fresh garlic cloves, minced
- 1 cup white wine
- 3/4 cup unsweetened almond milk or unsweetened coconut milk
- 1/4 cup homemade mayonnaise
- 2 Tbsps Dijon mustard
- a handful of fresh parsley, minced

Instructions

1. Heat a large skillet over medium heat and add in the oil and butter.
2. Meanwhile, season the chicken with sea salt, pepper, then lightly coat with flour.
3. Sauté your chicken until golden brown and cooked through, around 4-6 minutes on each side depending on the thickness of your breasts.
4. Set cooked chicken aside on a plate.
5. In that same preheated skillet add in the bacon and cook until it begins to crisp up nicely.
6. Once the bacon is almost done, add in the shallots and garlic into the skillet and sauté for 3 minutes.
7. Add in the wine to deglaze the pan, stirring all the tasty bits off the bottom and incorporating them into the wine. Simmer over medium heat for a few minutes until reduced by half.
8. Whisk in the milk, mayonnaise, and Dijon mustard, incorporating really well, then return your cooked chicken back to the skillet. Spoon sauce over chicken.
9. Cook the chicken for a couple of minutes more, just until hot and bubbly.
10. Garnish with parsley and serve while hot.
11. Enjoy!

Prep Time: 25 Minutes

Cook Time: 55 Minutes

Servings: 4

Ingredients

- 2 Tbsps avocado oil, divided
- 1 lb lean ground beef or bison
- 1/4 cup coconut aminos, tamari, Braggs liquid aminos, or low sodium soy sauce
- 1 Tbsp apple cider vinegar
- 3 fresh garlic cloves, minced
- 1-inch piece fresh ginger, grated
- 2 red bell peppers, seeded and diced
- 1-1/2 cups small chopped broccoli florets
- 4 cups cauliflower rice
- 3 large eggs, beaten
- 4 green onions, chopped
- 3 tsps sesame seeds

Instructions

1. Heat half of your oil in a large skillet or wok over medium-high heat. Stir fry the beef while mincing with a wooden spoon until golden and cooked through. Drain and discard any excess grease. Drizzle in the coconut aminos and apple cider vinegar into the beef, stir, then set beef aside on a plate.

2. Heat the remaining oil into the same skillet. Cook your garlic and ginger for 30 seconds. Stir in the bell pepper, and broccoli then stir fry for 2-3 minutes.

3. Add in your cauliflower rice and cook, stirring frequently for 3-4 minutes, or until

4. tender.

5. Push the veggies onto one side of your skillet. Pour the beaten eggs into the free space of the pan, and scramble until set;

6. Combine with the veggies. Return beef back into the pan and stir to combine and heat everything through.

7. Garnish with green onions and sesame seeds.

8. Enjoy!

Prep Time: 25 Minutes

Cook Time: 55 Minutes

Servings: 6

Ingredients

- 2 Tbsps olive oil, avocado oil, or ghee
- 2 lbs boneless, skinless chicken thighs, cut into large pieces
- sea salt and ground pepper, to taste
- 4 cloves fresh garlic, minced
- 4 large red sweet peppers, chopped into large pieces
- 2 sprigs of fresh rosemary
- 1 cup dry white wine
- 1 cup chicken broth
- a small handful of fresh chopped Italian parsley

Instructions

1. Heat your oil in a large skillet or Dutch oven over medium-high heat.

2. Add in the chicken pieces and sear for 5 minutes on all sides, or until golden brown. Season with sea salt and pepper. Your chicken doesn't need to be fully cooked through as we'll continue to cook it later on. Set aside.

3. In the same preheated skillet add in your garlic. Saute for 30 seconds, then add in the sweet peppers and rosemary sprigs. Cook, stirring frequently for 2-3 minutes. Pour in the wine and scrape the bottom of your pan to deglaze. Allow wine to reduce by half.

4. Return your chicken to the pan and stir in the broth.

5. Reduce your heat to low, cover, and simmer until the chicken it's fully cooked through, around 15 minutes.

6. Garnish with chopped fresh parsley and serve over cooked brown rice or quinoa if desired.

7. Enjoy!